UNDERSTANDING AND OVERCOMING DEPRESSION

BY

DR. J. T. MURRAY

In loving memory of my good friend Johnny White who lost his life due to depression.

PREFACE

With the increasing rate of suicide in the society due to individual going through different type of depression, this book helps identify the possible treatment and also help individuals through their recovery process

TABLE OF CONTENT

INTRODUTION

Depression has been a pandemic since the dawn of ages. Vivid pictures from historical and non-secular text describe sufferers of the sickness we tend to currently understand as depression. it exempt nobody irrespective of their race, sex, creed, religion, status and position. Its doubles fatal outcome "Suicide" is the third leading reason behind death.

This book mirrors the author belief that understanding depression is merely half the battle, taking personal responsibility for fighting the beast is equally necessary. The book additionally offers tips of fighting depression day by day.

CHAPTER ONE

WHAT IS DEPRESSION?

Being depressed typically appears like carrying a really serious burden; however you're not alone during this struggle. Several Americans suffer from some type of depression each year, creating it one in all the foremost common mental disorders within the country.

Gaining a deeper understanding of depression will facilitate begin the journey to recovery. Taking your time to find out additional concerning the causes and symptoms of depression can assist you greatly once it comes time to think about ways of treatment.

Depression is quite simply feeling unhappy. Everybody feels upset or wanton from time to time, however depression is additional serious. It's a mood disorder characterised by prolonged feelings of disappointment and loss of interest in daily activities. If these symptoms persist for a amount of a minimum of time period, it's thought of a depressive episode.

Depression (significant depressive disorder) is a prevalent and severe medical condition that has a negative impact on how you feel, thinking, and acting. Luckily, it can also be treated. Depression creates sorrow and/or loss of interest in once enjoyed operations. It can lead to a multitude of mental and physical issues and can diminish the capacity of a person to operate and operate.

Depression Is Different From Sadness or Grief / Bereavement

It is hard for a individual to endure the death of a loved one, the loss of a job or the termination of a partnership. Development in reaction to such circumstances is normal for emotions of sorrow or grief. Those who experience loss may often define them as "depressed," but being sad are not the same as being depressed. The grieving process is natural and special to each person, sharing some of the same depression characteristics. Intense sorrow and withdrawal from usual operations may require both grief and depression. In significant respects, they are also distinct:

1. Painful emotions come in waves in grief, often mixed with the deceased's

beneficial memories. Mood and/or interest (pleasure) are reduced for most of two weeks in major depression.

2. Usually, self-esteem is preserved in grief. Sensations of worthlessness and self-loathing are prevalent in significant depression.

CHAPTER TWO

CAUSES OF DEPRESSION

There are several causes of depression, as it depends on a combination of an individual's genetic makeup and environmental conditions. There are many factors to take into consideration:

1. family history of depression
2. Hormone change
3. Medication
4. Unrealistic educational, social, or family expectations will produce a powerful sense of rejection and might cause deep disappointment
5. traumatic events

CHAPTER THREE

TYPES OF DEPRESSION

1. Major Depressive Disorder (MDD)

They usually refer to major depressive disorder (MDD) when individuals use the word clinical depression. Major depressive disorder is a mood disorder with a number of main characteristics:

- Depressed mood
- Lack of interest in operations
- Usually enjoyed weight changes
- Changes in sleep
- fatigue
- feelings of worthlessness and guilt
- Difficulty to concentrate
- Death and suicide thoughts.

If an individual experiences most of these symptoms over a period of more than two weeks, they are often diagnosed with MDD.

Talk therapy can help. You'll meet with a mental health specialist who will help you find ways to manage your depression. Medications called

Antidepressants can also be useful.

When therapy and medication aren't working, two other options your doctor may suggest are:

- Electroconvulsive therapy (ECT)
- Repetitive trans cranial magnetic stimulation (RTMS)

ECT uses electrical pulses and RTMS uses a special kind of magnet to stimulate certain areas of brain activity. This helps the parts of your brain that control your mood work better.

2. Persistent Depressive Disorder.

Dysthymia, now referred to as persistent emotional disorder, refers to a kind of chronic depression gift for a lot of days than not for a minimum of 2 years. It is gentle, moderate, or severe.

- You may have symptoms such as:
- Change in your appetence (not ingestion enough or overeating)
- Sleep an excessive amount of or insufficient
- Lack of energy, or fatigue
- Low vanity
- Trouble concentrating or creating choices
- Feel hopeless

You may be treated with psychotherapy, medication, or a mixture of the 2.

3. Bipolar Disorder

Bipolar Disorder is a mood disorder characterised by periods of abnormally elevated mood called mania. These periods may be gentle (hypomania) or they'll be thus extreme on cause marked impairment with a personality's life, need hospitalization, or have an effect on a personality's sense of reality. The overwhelming majority of these with bipolar ill health even have episodes of major depression. Medication will facilitate bring your mood swings in check. Whether or not you are in an exceedingly high or an occasional amount, your doctor could recommend a mood stabilizer, such as lithium.

The FDA has approved three medicines to treat the depressed phase:

- Seroquel
- Latuda
- Olanzapine-fluoxetine combination

4. Seasonal Affective Disorder (SAD)

Seasonal affective disorder is a amount of major depression that the majority typically happens throughout the winter months, once the times grow short and you get less and fewer daylight. It generally goes away within the spring and summer.

If you've got unhappy, antidepressants will facilitate. Thus will light-weight medical aid. You'll have to sit down before of a special bright light-weight box for concerning 15-30 minutes daily.

SAD is a lot of common in so much northern or so much southern regions of the earth.

5. Peripartum (Postpartum) Depression

Women have major depression within the weeks and months once giving birth could have peripartum depression. Medicine medication will facilitate equally to treating major depression that's unrelated to giving birth.

6. Premenstrual Dysphoric Disorder (PMDD)

Women with PMDD have depression and alternative symptoms at the beginning of their period.

Besides feeling depressed, you will additionally have:

- Extreme fatigue
- Feeling unhappy, hopeless, or self-critical
- Severe feelings of stress or anxiety
- Mood swings, typically with bouts of crying
- Irritability
- Inability to concentrate
- Food cravings or binging

7. Atypical Depression

Do you expertise signs of depression (such as gluttony, sleeping and excessive amount of extreme sensitivity to rejection) however end up suddenly perking up in face of a positive event?

It is really a lot of common than the name may imply. Not like different kinds of depression, folks with atypical depression might respond higher to a kind of antidepressant drug referred to as a monoamine oxidase inhibitor (MAO).☐☐

CHAPTER FOUR

COPING WITH

DEPRESSION

You can't just "snap out of it" when you are depressed, but this tips can help bring you to the path of recovery.

Why is managing depression therefore difficult?

Depression drains your energy, hope, and drive, creating it tough to require the steps that may assist you to feel higher. Sometimes, simply pondering the items you ought to do to feel higher, like workout or outlay time with friends, will appear exhausting or not possible to place into action.

While convalescent from depression isn't fast or simple, you do have more control than you realize —even if your depression is severe and pig-headedly persistent. The secret is to begin little and build from there

By taking the subsequent tiny however positive steps day by day, you'll before long elevate the serious fog of depression and end up feeling happier, healthier, and a lot of hopeful once more.

1. Reach out and stay connected
   - Look for support from those who cause you to feel safe and cared for
   - Try to maintain with social activities notwithstanding you don't want it
   - Join a support group for depression.
   - Care for a pet

2. Do things that make you feel good

3. Eat a healthy, depression-fighting diet

- Don't skip meals
- Minimize sugar and refined carbs
- Boost your B vitamins
- Boost your mood with foods rich in omega-3 fatty acids

4. Get a daily dose of daylight

Sunlight will facilitate boost monoamine neurotransmitter levels and improve your mood. Whenever doable, get outside throughout daytime and expose yourself to the sun for a minimum of quarter-hour each day by taking a walk, exercising outside, opening blinds at home and workplace and sitting close to the window.

5. Stop negative thoughts.

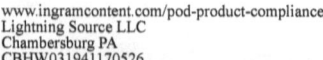